It's Probably Nothing . . .*

*Or How I Learned to Stop Worrying
and Love My Implants*

Micki Myers

Simon & Schuster

New York   London   Toronto   Sydney   New Delhi

Simon & Schuster
1230 Avenue of the Americas
New York, NY 10020

First Simon & Schuster hardcover edition October 2013

SIMON & SCHUSTER and colophon are registered trademarks of Simon & Schuster, Inc.

For information about special discounts for bulk purchases, please contact Simon & Schuster Special Sales at 1-866-506-1949 or business@simonandschuster.com.

The Simon & Schuster Speakers Bureau can bring authors to your live event. For more information or to book an event contact the Simon & Schuster Speakers Bureau at 1-866-248-3049 or visit our website at www.simonspeakers.com.

Designed by Ruth Lee-Mui

Manufactured in the United States of America

1   3   5   7   9   10   8   6   4   2

Library of Congress Cataloging-in-Publication Data

Myers, Micki, 1967–
It's probably nothing, or, How I learned to stop worrying and love my implants / Micki Myers. —First Simon & Schuster hardcover edition.
pages cm
1. Myers, Micki, 1967– —Poetry. 2. Cancer in women—Poetry. 3. Cancer—Patients—Poetry. I. Title.

PS3613.Y474I87 2013
811'.6—dc23   2013008888

ISBN 978-1-5011-8703-2
ISBN 978-1-4767-1276-5 (ebook)

*For my dear Poppo, who wished a wish
no parent should ever have come true, and
Lucia, Javier, and Matthew,
who are my whole world, with love.*

"Don't worry—
eighty percent of these biopsies
come back negative."
—*Nurse, day one*

Contents

Stage IV   97

It's Probably Nothing . . .*

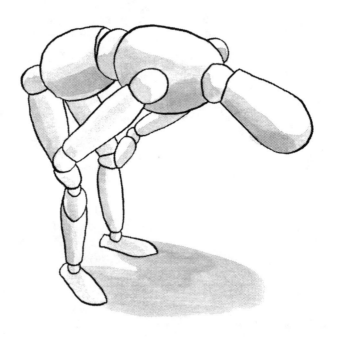

Oh Fuck! I Have Cancer!

There is no book in the library
titled *Oh Fuck! I Have Cancer!*
because if there was, I'd have
checked it out. Instead, there is
a wide selection of medical texts
and survivor accounts and memorials
and "helpful" hints featuring
older women who are active
in their church who have
lots of cats and husbands
who held them while they puked.
There is no book that will tell me
if silicone boobs wobble during sex
or if reconstructed nipples chafe.

In short, the really useful stuff.

Publishers offering HUGE advances,
library acquisitions officers, listen up:
a book titled *Oh Fuck! I Have Cancer!*
will be the first thing a newly diagnosed woman
will reach for every time, I don't care
how many cats she has.

Seriously.
Call me.

Stage I

Dream a Little Dream of Me

for Tim

It begins with a dream.
You were holding your breast, he says,

and so I do
and there it is,

far to the right,
a lump the size of a small grape.

Or a large peanut. Or a cranberry.
Or a cherry pit, or a bean.

Despite all the food analogies,
I've suddenly lost my appetite.

No Way! *Way.*

You only find out afterwards
that by the time you can feel
the lump yourself, it's already
been there for about ten years.

Don't Waffle About:
Get a Mammogram!

Despite what everyone tells you,
a regular mammogram is not the worst thing
that can happen to your boobs.

When the plates squeeze each one flat
in order to peer inside,
do not think of where the insides go—

whether, like a waffle iron
filled with too much batter,
it might all leak out the sides.

Don't worry: they bounce right back.
It's the post-biopsy mammograms
that you want to avoid,

because they hurt so much,
the only thing you'll wish
you could associate a waffle iron with

is breakfast.

It's Probably Nothing . . .

No, actually,
it's *everything*.

I know you mean
to be reassuring,

but the only thing
"nothing" refers to right now

is what else
is on my mind.

A Living Wage

The nurse who gets to call you
with the results of your first biopsy
doesn't get paid enough.

She gives you a list of
surgical oncologists
you have to call right away.
Like *today*.

I don't care what she makes,
it's not enough.

What to Expect When You're Expecting to Hear You Have Cancer

Congratulations!
Start saying your goodbyes!

The tumor is the size of a grapefruit/cantaloupe/
    basketball—
and getting bigger every day!

That's really inconvenient of you.

You have a ninety percent chance of survival.
Oh, hang on—that was upside down.
I mean you have a six percent chance of survival.
Oops.

Wow—it's hard to believe you're still alive!
How are you feeling?

We've never seen anything like that before.
We're not sure what it is exactly, but it'll have to come out.
Somehow.

Oh good—we've been waiting for someone
we can practice this experimental surgery on.

Man, I wouldn't want to be you.

Look: prosthetics nowadays have come a long way.
Almost no one will be able to tell.

You know what they say: life begins at forty!

You always wanted a breast reduction—
now you can get one for free!

The Bionic Woman was sexy, right?
Right?

It's not that bad: it's not like anyone
but your husband gets to see your breasts anyway.

Are you going to lose one? Or both? Or just part of one?
You don't want to end up lopsided.

Seriously, wigs are hip right now.
And it's nearly Halloween, so they'll be cheap!

Just think of the money you'll save
on bras and haircuts!

Great! This is your chance to get some tits
you can actually be proud of!

Woo-hoo! Implants!
All your friends will be so jealous.

There's this brand-new drug which has shown great
    promise in mice,
but we'd like to test it out on a human. Wanna try?

Nipples are so overrated.

Treat it like an adventure. Like a really horrifying, painful,
scary, expensive adventure people go on in documentaries.

We can't treat that.

Does your insurance cover this?

Scars heal. I mean the internal scars are worse than the
    external ones.
I mean you'll be scarred, sure, but the scars
will be on the inside, so no one will know.

Can I have your shoes and jewelry and purses?
And that really pretty dress I borrowed that one time?

Well, my mother/sister/aunt/coworker/that celebrity had
    it and they're fine.
Nothing to worry about. And my aunt had it twice!

What if it's spread?
Already?

Do you need a tissue?

Are you sitting down?

Bedside Manners

Dr. K stands beside me
as I lie on the exam table,
quietly reaches out to touch my breast
and closes his eyes.

He keeps them closed as he moves
his hands, caressing, softly pressing,
making gentle circles, carefully teasing up
and pinching my nipple, rolling it between his fingers.

It's the most sensual time I've had on my back in years
until he breaks the silence and says
"I'm afraid we're not going to be able to save it."
"The whole thing?" I ask, all trembly-voiced.

"Yes," he replies, "I'm very sorry."
I promptly start crying.
I can hear every Momma everywhere
saying the same old thing:

If you let a boy feel you up on a first date,
mark my words—it'll only end in tears.

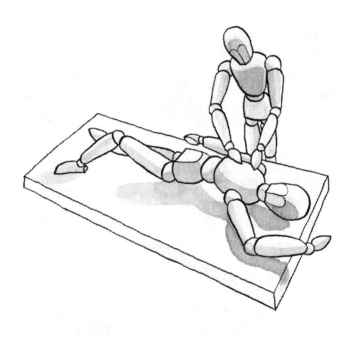

Say Wha?

A health history questionnaire
for the High Risk Breast and
Ovarian Cancer Center asks
"Have you recently felt
worried or anxious
for no reason?"

Are they kidding?
No reason?

Mind Over Matter

The surgical oncologist
wants to bombard me with radiation
even though the data says
that at my age, the long-term harm
it *would* cause is greater than
the short-term benefits
it *might* provide.

"Thanks, but I'll take my chances,"
I tell him. I get the feeling
he doesn't like it when patients read data.
He's all about protocol,
and he's not convinced.

"You don't want to wonder
if every headache you get
is a brain tumor," he says.

Gee, thanks.
I've already got a damn headache
just thinking about it.

You Want the Good News
or the Bad News?

When I go in for my test results,
the genetics counselor greets me
with a big smile and says,
"What do *you* think I'm going to say?"

After I was diagnosed,
my uncle said, "Oh, breast cancer—
every woman in our family gets that."

Come again?

Turns out he's right.

I look down at my lap.
"Blue genes," I say.

Tie a Pink Ribbon Around
the Old Oak Tree

When I look up all my female ancestors on Ancestry.com
to see if the rumors are true
—that they all had breast cancer—
I see they're all marked with a green leaf
instead of a pink ribbon,
which would be far more useful.

Apparently they all died of Dutch elm disease.

617delT Walks into a Bar

Mitzvah somewhere in northern Europe
and leaves behind an invisible gift
that will keep giving for generations to come.
Three thousand years later, it's still showing up,
an uninvited guest telling people
they won't be getting any older.

Stereotactic Core Biopsy
Black and Blues

To put me at ease, the doctor says

Simple, simple.
We just take some tissue samples
guided by X-ray. Nothing to it.
Go home same day. Small bandage.
We use lidocaine shot, easy-peasy.
You won't feel a thing.
You just lie there. Go to sleep!
Fifteen, twenty minutes, tops.

The doctor is a liar liar pants on fire.

In fact, this procedure involves
lying belly-down on the table
with your boob hanging through a hole
and squashed between two plates,
head twisted to one side,
while a machine inserts a hollow needle
as thick as a pencil into your breast
to extract samples.

Halfway through,
the lidocaine wears off.

Too bad, too bad,
the doctor says.
Very bad if you pass out.
Must stay awake.

It's the first honest thing
he's uttered all day.

Muzak

The hospital atrium's automatic piano
is treating us to a spirited rendition
of the Elton John catalogue
at double speed and out of key.

There's nothing like a wobbly
"I'm Still Standing" to give you the impression
the tests aren't going to come back good.

Double Whammy

It's bad enough coming to terms
with the thought of losing one breast,
let alone two. But the reality facing
the prospects of the healthy one
doesn't appear to leave much to consider.

First, there's the surgery
to lift it to match the implant,
then there's the chance
the cancer will return
and ravage it anyway.

I decide on the *double whammy*
—one breast to save my life now,
and one breast to save it in the future.
It's a gamble, but the odds
I've escaped the genetic bullet
that threatens to kill me
are pretty slim.

Of course, with no boobs,
I'll make a smaller target,
especially in profile.

So there's that.

Agent Provocateur

Prior to surgery, I spend some quality time
at the sexiest, most expensive lingerie store I can find,
trying on outfits so that I can have memories
of what could have been. I hope the salesgirl
can't tell I have no intention of ever buying any of it.
It's an exercise in wistfulness, hooks and eyes,
black ribbon, leather and lace.
Not bad for thirty-nine, I think.

Two years later I return with brand-new 36Bs.
It's astonishing how much better
everything fits (and looks)
when you have the boobs of a nineteen-year-old.

Body Piercing

Prep for the biopsy involves
injecting a radioactive dye into the breast
so that its path can be traced
to the sentinel lymph node in the armpit,
which is then easily located and removed
to see if the cancer has spread.

When I say "injected into the breast," I mean
a nurse rolls up a towel, asks me to bite down on it,
("Trust me about this," she says),
then pushes a large needle into my nipple.

Into, not *through*.

Through ain't got shit on this.

Sentinel Node Biopsy Lament

No one tells you that having a lymph-node biopsy
will rob you of your ability to make pastry.

That even if it looks like your arm is normal,
in fact you cannot rely on it to hold a kettle,

fetch a bottle of milk from the fridge.
You will get used to dropping stuff.

You will become a poor typist,
looking up to find gibberish on the screen.

Forget handwriting. Forget drawing.
Forget knitting. Forget "ticklish."

Forget the guitar, the piano, the flute.
Forget manicures and tattoos.

Yeah, I know what you're thinking.
Forget *that*, too.

Sadenfreude

When two people compete
to see whose ailments are

more grievous, often starting out
with minor annoyances

(broken nail; varicose veins)
which are one-upped

until one of them says
"Yeah, but I have cancer."

Freefalling

My friend, trying to put
a good spin on it, tells me
that at least my boobs
will never droop when I get old.

Neither one of us
states the obvious:
that the rest of me,
however,
will.

You Can Never Be Too Rich
or Too Thin?

The plastic surgeon wants to have a look
to see what kind of reconstruction is possible.
While I am standing there in nothing but my panties,
she turns me this way and that,
pinching a bit of flesh here and there.
"There's not a lot of you to work with,"
she says, clearly disappointed.

Most women are happy to go for
the upgrade: the excess flab moved around
for a tummy tuck and boob job all in one.

So much for being fit and forty.

Better to have let yourself go a bit,
it turns out. Or a *lot*, if you want
really impressive knockers.

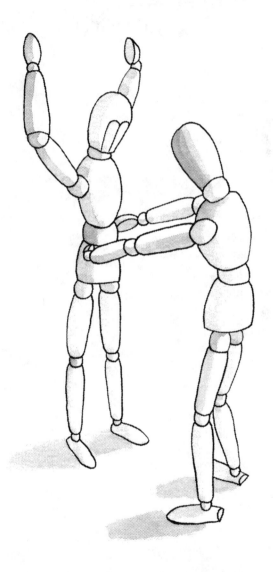

I've Got a Lovely Bunch of Coconuts

The physician's assistant hands me
a manila envelope containing
before and after pictures of women
with the sort of implants I'm going for.

It's a showcase of the plastic surgeon's best work.

Everyone looks like they've been
made out of clay by a child,
with two nubby mounds
sticking out of their chests
and no nipples. It's horrifying.

I slip the pictures back in
out of modesty or embarrassment
and thank the lady
and drive away.

B31-3 Rosette Royal with
a Little SR512 Fruit Punch

It occurs to me
that I ought to make a record
of my nipple color
for when the reconstruction team
make me new ones.
I do not want to go through all this
and end up with orange headlamps.

This is how I come to be standing
at the bathroom window
holding paint samples
from Home Depot
up to my chest,
hoping the neighbors
don't notice.

You Can't Take It with You

The night before surgery,
my first, scheduled to last
at least six hours,
it occurs to me
that I ought to leave
some instructions,
just in case.

I look around at all my stuff
and realize I don't really care
who gets what, and just leave
one small sentimental thing
to each child, more a gesture
than anything else.

It's a sobering exercise.

Then I go and kiss their foreheads
as they sleep, as I have done
every night of their lives.
They do not know I do this.
It doesn't matter.

Stage II

What a Racket

I awake from surgery,
a nurse checks me over,
removes the catheter
(deep breath!), shows me
the button for the morphine drip,
and tells me to let her know
if there's anything I need.
Then she walks away.

My throat is parched,
too dry to speak, so I try to lift
my arm to get her attention
for a glass of water,
but she's sitting at her station
gossiping on the phone,
facing the other direction.

It's a very long conversation—
I can see the clock
on the recovery room wall
perfectly well.

I think I might have survived the surgery
only to die of thirst.

And for this they charge
my HMO as unholy a sum
as you can possibly imagine.

The Penny Drops

You think it's just going to be
your chest that's messed up
after surgery, but when
you try to move, you realize
that the lymph-node dissection
has rendered your right arm useless.
You think *move*
but it doesn't.

When you're alone
in your hospital room
and the phone rings,
all you can do
is stare at it.

"I'll be right there," you say,
not moving.

Should you need a nurse,
you have no way of pushing the call button,
which has thoughtfully been placed
to the right of the bed.

The phone rings again.
"Coming!" you say.

This strikes you as very funny indeed
until you realize you have to pee.

Penicillin

amoxicillin, cephalexin
erythromycin, clarithromycin, azithromycin
ciprofloxacin, levofloxacin, ofloxacin
trimethoprim, tetracycline, doxycycline
gentamicin, tobramycin

These are the gods you pray to,
hoping not to fall out of favor
by worshipping at their altar too much.
For when a god turns his back,
you are thus smited with hives and rashes,
wheezing, swelling, and death.

A color-coded plastic wristband
lets the hospital staff know
which is your savior,
and which will speed you
to your maker.

Pathological

I'm used to thinking of margins
as edges, thin spaces that form a boundary
from one area to another, marked
by a thin red line, as on a ruled page.

How close you conform to the margin
says a lot about your personality—
you either stray further and further from it
as you work your way down, less conscious
of the space in which your thought is contained,
or you remain tight upon it, ever aware of its pull.

I always liked marginalia, the scribblings
that readers leave behind to mark a text,
until now—when anything but clean margins
could spell a death sentence writ in flesh.

Acronymious

The hospital's parting gifts include:
a range of plastic breathing instruments
to help strengthen my collapsed lung
and prevent me from getting pneumonia;
some bandages; a cartload of painkillers;
a mastectomy bra; and a case of
methicillin-resistant *Staphylococcus aureus*,
the dreaded MRSA, a staph infection
which threatens to kill me dead.

They give it an acronym not because
its name is hard to pronounce,
but because acronyms sound relatively benign,
a good PR ploy given that MRSA
is resistant to modern antibiotics.

Ancient antibiotics however,
such as honey and silver,
work very well.
When I suggest this remedy,
the nurses just LOL.

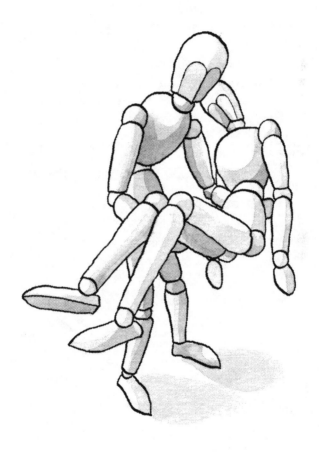

On the Hospital Menu: Takeout

On the morning I'm due to be discharged
from the hospital, one woman, then another
pops her head around my door
to take a peek at me. One of them
exclaims "Oh my God! She's tiny!"

I know I haven't eaten the food,
but I can't have lost *that* much weight
since being admitted.

When she comes back later
with a post-mastectomy camisole
with pockets for polyester stuffing
"to approximate the look of real breasts
under clothing" (a gift from the hospital
as consolation for what I've lost),
she tells me they had a hard time
finding one my size (XS).

When I leave, they can only find
a double-wide wheelchair
for me to sit in, compounding
that shrunken feeling.

It turns out my room was on the floor
reserved for women going in for
stomach-stapling surgery.

You Can't Make a Silk Purse
out of a Sow's Ear

Having a skin-sparing bilateral mastectomy
means you have a lot of spare skin
hanging around on your chest
like two pursed lips.

The surgical drains clipped
to the waistband of your pants
feel like grenades.

It's easier to stick to similes
instead of committing your fate to metaphor,
because it's hard to believe
that what you see in the mirror
will ever again be something
you could tuck some spare change in
when out on the town.

Wussy

My plastic surgeon is a petite woman
    whose lack of stature and muscle mass
        is more than made up for in attitude.

When it's time to take the surgical drains out
    she's all business. "Deep breath," she says,
        then yanks.

The ones she pulls from my armpits
    aren't that bad; after all, I can't feel anything
        as they've severed all the nerves.

It's the one embedded eight inches in my chest
    that makes me scream when she pulls.
        "Don't be a wuss," she chastises.

I shoot her a look, you know the one.
    But if I'm being honest,
        it's pretty good advice, all in all.

Air Re-conditioning

Surprisingly, the biggest difference
you notice is something you
never noticed before:
walking into a supermarket
and not having your nipples
get hard from the blast of cool air.

You'll never ever feel that again.

You never thought it possible
to be jealous of the women
you usually see in there,
but now you are.

We spend all of our lives
hiding our nipples
as if having them on display
would mean they'd get pinched
by someone who wants to know
how ripe they are.

"It Costs a Lot of Money to Look This Cheap"

—*Dolly Parton*

I never wore high heels
or short-shorts
or fancy knickers
or mascara
or flashy earrings
until I had no breasts.

Some hooker I'd make.

Spit or Swallow?

Prep for the CT scan requires that I drink two giant
    bottles
of barium sulfate solution,

or what the nurse gleefully refers to
as "banana shake."

This is because the only flavor they have is banana.
And because she shakes it.

Beyond that, there is no earthly resemblance
to a shake of any kind, banana or not.

It's nothing like milk, and tastes like paint.
I have an hour. I am advised to pace myself.

With fifteen minutes left and an entire container still to go,
I visit the bathroom and flush the whole thing.

Back in the waiting room,
I pretend to finish it off with a flourish.

Oh come on: I know I'm not the only girl
who's ever faked it.

Disabled Driver

I am pretty sure that the DMV would prefer
that drivers have full range of motion
in their arms when operating a moving vehicle.

How else am I going to get to
my physical therapy appointment
if I don't drive?

Every week, they measure
incremental gains—a centimeter here,
a bit more grip there.

By the end of the first month,
I can even use my right arm to help steer
by leaning my shoulder into the wheel.

I'd love to be able to park
in one of the disabled spots,
but as a recent amputee

with half the use of my left arm,
and none of my right one,
I am not disabled *enough*
to score a windshield sticker.

Stage III

Biohazard

Have you been feeling run down because you've been told you have cancer? Have you lost your spark? Do your loved ones complain about your prospects? Do you often feel apprehensive about your upcoming surgeries and worry that you will lose the use of your arms? Does the suffix "-ectomy" fill you with dread? Do tears come all too easily? Have you lost your sense of humor? Are you depressed?

If you've experienced any of these symptoms, then ask your doctor about Adriamycin. It can help keep you alive. And that's a good thing. Combined with a number of other chemotherapeutic agents, a program of radical surgery, radiation, and ten years of tamoxifen, it has been shown to be ninety percent effective in keeping you alive for at least five whole years. And as you know all too well, when it comes to cancer, percentages are everything.

Adriamycin is not tolerated by everyone; alert a health professional if you develop uncontrollable vomiting, drastic weight loss, severe alopecia, red urine, runny nose, reduced sex drive, extreme fatigue, muscle wasting, severe blood disorders, or sudden heart failure. Adriamycin can and will cause tissue damage if not administered properly. If you notice blistering at the injection site or your arm falls off, notify your doctor. People

taking Adriamycin have been known to die suddenly. If you die
suddenly, seek medical help immediately by calling 911.

Do not take Adriamycin if you have had a recent heart attack,
have heart disease, liver problems, an infection caused by a
fungus, are pregnant or could become pregnant, are producing
milk or breast-feeding, have iffy blood or broke-ass bone mar-
row. Do not take Adriamycin if you have a fear of needles and/
or hospital settings. Do not take Adriamycin if you are scared
of sudden death.

Don't become a statistic: ask your doctor about Adriamy-
cin (doxorubicin) today.

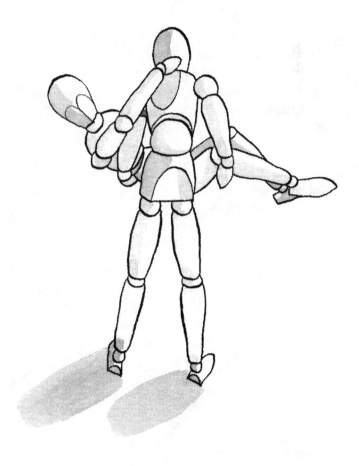

Wigging Out

"You'll need one of these," the nurse practitioner says,
and hands me a catalogue filled with the head
of a beatific-looking young woman of about twenty-two
with perfect makeup and very white teeth
modeling hundreds of different wigs.

A lot of them are gray or white
and look incongruous on so young a girl.
They all have names like *The Audrey* and *The Anne*.

Their real name, however,
is written on the prescription:
Total Cranial Prosthesis.

That Old Red Devil Called Love

The Adriamycin comes in a sealed bag
emblazoned with a giant skull and crossbones,
as if its syrupy redness in the syringe didn't look
scary enough. Everything it touches
needs to be sealed back in and disposed of
in the toxic waste container after it's been
pushed into my vein.
The chemo nurse wears two sets of thick
latex gloves to touch me while my arm
remains bare, carefully checking my
ID band twice so as not to kill me
by accident with someone else's dose.

The devil really does wear a disguise.

And yes, they don't call it what it really is,
which is liquid mustard gas—
something they don't generally advertise.

Seeing Red

The dye in the Adriamycin is so strong
that it turns your urine crimson.
"That's how we know it's working!"

I'm glad they warned me about this
because otherwise I might fear
I was dying.

Honeymoon

The first two weeks you think *WTF?*
That wasn't so bad, I'm gonna sail through this
like nobody's business, and besides,
I feel so fit and healthy!
I will be the exception to the rule
and confound all my doctors and impress
all my friends and woo-hoo! Look! I can eat
no problemo, I can do three hours of
backbreaking work in the garden
and still have energy left over to play
with the kids and obviously I'm not losing
my hair because it's all still here and
I'm gonna sail through this easy-peasy—

and then day 17 arrives
and that cruise you were taking
hits an iceberg just like that—
and instead of dancing a jig
you're clinging to a flotation device
that's just sprung a leak.

Short Back and Sides

The razor makes a slight hiss
as it glides over your scalp,
one hand feeling the way
to find where the stubble is.

Although it's something you dreaded
having to do, it actually feels very sensual,
a pleasant surprise.

You wonder whether men
get the same thrill polishing their heads
when they too lose their locks.

You lather up your face,
just for the hell of it,
and shave the way you've seen them do.

Standing there—bald, flat-chested,
wearing a beard of foam—
you realize you've never felt more
like a woman in your whole life.

Blessed Are the Children

For my five-year-old daughter
looks inquisitively at me
in the bathroom
and then at herself.

For my three-year-old son says
"Mummy, I love your bald head!"

Opportunity Knocks!

Now that the chemo
has taken away all
the hair *down there*,
I'm finally able
to live out my fantasy
of being a porno model.

It's not like they have
boob-surgery scars
or wear wigs, right?

Right.

Escapism

In the waiting room,
you sit through
the inescapable drone
of the very dregs of what
daytime TV can offer—
the women's chat shows,
the cooking shows,
the soap operas.

It's enough to make you
think survival
is overrated.

Teaching on Percocets

Because I am a tough motherfucker
(and also have student loans to pay),
I maintain my teaching schedule through chemo.

It's not bad: a couple of three-hour classes
once a week at the university.

The first week of class I still have my hair.
The second, I do not.

Some explaining has to be done.

I tell them not to panic,
but I'm really very high,
and that because I have no immune system,
should anyone give me a cold
I'm likely to drop dead,
possibly on the spot.

*   *   *

I wish I could tell you all about
how wild and crazy it is giving lectures
while amped up on serious painkillers,

and how much fun my students had
taking advantage of my compromised state,
or about how I eased my grading burden
by giving them all A's for putting up with me,

but after that second week, everything's a blur.

I could have been conducting an orchestra
of clowns riding unicorns for all I know.

And that's probably what it looked like, too.

Don't Call Us—We'll Call You!

Contrary to popular belief,
you can't catch cancer
over the phone.

Still, this doesn't stop
people from not calling you
to see if you're still alive.

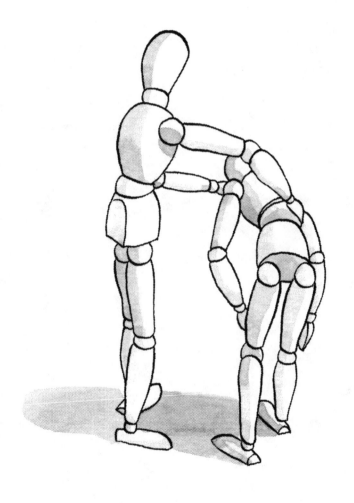

Neupogen

The only shot that hurts so bad
it makes you wish
you'd been shot instead.

THC, TLC, TCB

Marinol is a drug that has been developed
to replicate the wondrous effects
of plain old weed.

It can only be prescribed
if all other available antiemetics
have failed to relieve your life-threatening nausea,
and then, it can only be administered
in a hospital setting with careful monitoring
by trained staff in case you take a funny turn.

No one appears to know about it,
which is perhaps the point.

But it only comes in pill form,
so you have to swallow it,
which is near impossible
when you're puking,
and even if you manage to keep it down
it takes a long time to kick in.

A puff on a marijuana cigarette,
on the other hand,
works immediately.

They try to give it to kids
on the children's chemo ward
so that they can eat.

Because God forbid you give
dying children a smoke
to relieve their pain.

As far as I'm concerned,
you can give children on chemo
any damn thing they please.

The Funnies

Good weed is wasted on chemo.

When you get the munchies,
all you can manage to get down
is a tablespoon of rice.

When you get horny,
you're too toxic to touch.

Lethargy is a step up from "normal,"
and you're paranoid about everything already.

It does allow you to find all of this
terribly amusing, however.

Sorry to Be So Blunt

Oddly enough, while most of my time on chemo
is a giant blur (blame chemo brain),
I can remember clear as if it were yesterday
being at my most skeletal, and needing to eat,

trying to roll a pre-dinner joint,
leaning on the kitchen counter
to hold myself up, and producing
something as wide around as a tampon,

the papers barely stuck together,
fumbling to strike a match
(the coordination and strength required
to flick a lighter utterly beyond me),

and sucking deep from the end not on fire,
inhaling crumbled leaf, sticks and seeds,
choking mildly and spitting,
then sliding from the counter to the floor,

where I lay in blissful peace,
giggling like an idiot, while my children
watched from the dinner table.
"Something's wrong with Mummy," my daughter said.

20-Gauge

Not the shotgun: the IV needle.

That's what the nurses claim they use
to shoot the chemo up with,
but it isn't.
They used 12-gauge on me.
I know this because I kept one of them.

The difference between being shot
with a 12-gauge instead of a 20-gauge
is akin to a scratch and
getting your face blown off.

Sometimes it takes six or seven tries
for the nurse to hit the vein right,
working her way up your arm
so the drugs don't leak out of the holes
she's left behind.

When your arm's all used up
they use your palm instead.
They don't tell you this
in the helpful cancer books.

If needles make you queasy,
don't get cancer.
Opt for something else.

I saw a woman pass out once,
dropping like a dead deer to the floor,
thump—just like that.

And she wasn't even the one
they were aiming at.
She was just there with a friend
for support.

Day Spa

The best things about the chemo ward
are the blanket-warming oven
and the heat lamp mounted
above every recliner.

If you close your eyes and ears and nose and mouth
you can pretend you're at a fancy spa
except that when you leave,
your skin is as crappy as it ever was
and none of your nails are done.

"Next week, ladies!" you warble
as you do your best to sashay out.

Hair Today, Gone Tomorrow Haiku

Folks think the worst thing
about chemo is losing
your hair. It isn't.

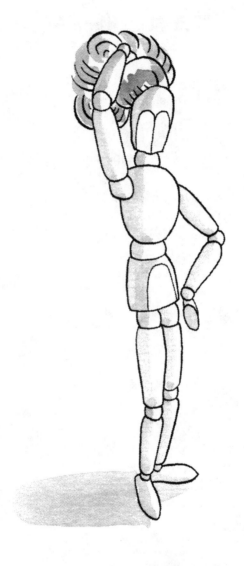

Yew Tree, How Scary Thou Art

My house, like many others in Pittsburgh,
is surrounded by yews, planted in some 1950s
misguided ornamental gardening frenzy.
Most have grown so large as to obscure
the ground-floor windows completely.

Long a feature of churchyards,
where they were planted to discourage
farm animals from grazing
amid the gravestones,
every part of the yew is utterly toxic
except for the bright red berries
which look very poisonous indeed.

Tamoxifen, the miracle drug
that helps prevent metastasis,
is made from yews.

The irony is not lost on me
that every time I warn my kids against
eating the tempting fruit,
it is this tree of death
that's keeping me alive.

Tragicomic

Your first several attempts
at drawing on eyebrows.

With practice, you settle
on merely dramatic.

Falsies

If you thought applying false eyelashes was hard
when you had real ones to guide you,
try doing it without.

No Such Thing as a Free Lunch

In the chemo room at noon,
a woman wheels a food cart around
asking if any of us want something to eat.

It's a white paper bag containing
a sandwich, a squeeze pouch of mayo,
a cookie, an apple, and a can of ginger ale.

Most people are attached to that drip
all day long.

No one ever takes a bag.

It's not that we're not hungry,
it's just that it's hospital food,
and reminds you of being sick.

When you're dying of cancer,
the last thing you want is a healthy,
well-balanced lunch.

How about a sizzling steak and fries?
How about cupcakes?
How about a juicy peach

in the middle of winter,
washed down with a glass of champagne?

I nickname the chemo ward "Death Row,"
and daydream I'm ordering up my last meal.

For all I know, it could be.

Tangled Up in You

Wearing high heels to your chemo appointments
as a *fuck you* to having lost most of your dignity
by being there in the first place
is awesome and everything
until you become entangled in the lines
hanging from your portable IV stand
as you dash to the bathroom
when the diarrhea hits.

I'd Raise Eyebrows,
If Anyone Had Them

It doesn't need to be Halloween
for you to wear your best
skull and crossbones T-shirt
to get your chemo.

Every day with cancer
is trick or treat.

Getting Lippy

When you're bald,
you fear people staring at you,
but they don't; most folks look away.

To draw attention from the stocking cap
in place of your hair,
you begin wearing bright red lipstick.

You imagine this looks *chic*,
like someone from a fashion magazine,
especially since you're now a size two.

What you fail to appreciate
is that it is your mind (and not just your body)
that has been ravaged by drugs,
and that your imagination

has yet to catch up.

Baa Baa Black Sheep

You think it's the chemo drug that
is most likely to kill you, but it isn't:
it's an allergic reaction to the solvent it comes in.

It's not the cancer that kills you either—
it's the damage it inflicts on everything around it
that does you in.

Infections are called "opportunistic,"
because they are smarter than you
and exploit your weaknesses
such as your lack of an immune system.

They're wolves in sheep's clothing
who find you because you stick out
like a sore thumb with your false hair,
mutton dressed as lamb,

bleating your woes
every chance you get.

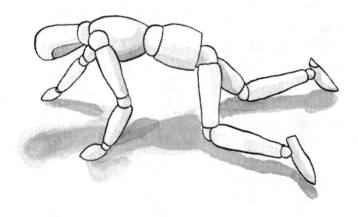

Make Mine a Double

Carol, my chemo nurse,
is exactly what
a chemo nurse should be:
careful, cheerful, funny,
kind, and competent.
She makes sure to get
the IV in properly,
gets me a warm blanket,
always cross-checks
my wristband to make sure
that the stuff in the drip bags
is actually for me.

She never hooks me up
with a straight vodka, though,
even when I remind her
it all looks the same,
and no one would know.

Magic Swizzle

Cancer's almost worth it for the drugs.
Or just the names of the drugs.

I thought this was a nickname
for what they had prescribed me

for a sore throat, a bit of jargon
they used for fun, but the label

on the bottle said *Magic Swizzle*
and the pharmacist winked

when he handed it to me, saying
"Lucky you—this stuff is *the shit*."

Mental Floss

They say that to forestall
the detrimental effects
of the dreaded "chemopause,"
it's good to take up
brain-stimulating activities
to keep sharp.

I can do the *Nation*
Cryptic Crossword just fine.

It's where I parked my car
or what day of the week it is
that stumps me.

Wastoid

All your life you're told
not to waste things,
and to feel guilty if you do.

When you kill an opponent
in a video game,
you waste them quickly.

Me, on the other hand—
I'm wasting away slowly
one cell at a time.

Hospital-Grade Benadryl

The first few weeks in the chemo room,
you wonder how anyone can let themselves
lie there in full view
fast asleep with their mouths
gaping open, snoring, even.
Have they no self-respect?

Then it's week 25
and you awaken to find
your tongue dry, hanging out
half an hour after
the drip has finished,
and Carol, your chemo nurse,
tells you she didn't want
to disturb you, you looked like
you needed the rest.

You're so grateful
you could cry.

Black Humor

There is a lot to be thankful that you forget.
The smell of chemo, the nausea.
The dread of going through it yet another week.

Cramming down bagfuls of Corn Pops
before a treatment, knowing you have to bulk up
as much as you can before even the *thought*
of swallowing makes you sick.

But there is one thing I'd like to remember:
it's a joke about an old couple involving a twist,
a double entendre or a misunderstanding,
and the punch line is so filthy, so unspeakably rude,
that you have to tell it in a whisper.

But I forgot *it* too.

It was my favorite joke to tell as we lay there
hooked up to our poison drips,
bald, half-dead skeletons laughing so hard
we kicked our blankets off.

It sounded like we were twisting the keys
and punching the gas, our gasps a loud throttle
trying to pump our rusty old engines back into life.

Death and Taxol

Ben Franklin knew a thing or two
about heeding tingling feelings,
but he never had to put up with
the long-nerve neuropathy
caused by paclitaxel,
the eleventh dose of which
is enough for me.

They recommend twelve.

I can no longer feel my fingers,
fumble everything,
want to quit while there's still
a chance I'll live to type again.
I'm not certain I'll beat death,
but am sure I'll lose my touch.

I'm a writer, I say to my oncologist,
half shrug, half plea,
holding up my hands.

She says OK.

Still Here

One day, after you've been
wrestling around on the floor
laughing with your children,
wearing your figure-hugging top
designed for a fifteen-year-old
that really shows off your new cleavage,
in your size two jeans (thanks, chemo!),

it occurs to you
that they're a whole year older
than they were a year ago.

And so are you.

Stage IV

Recovery, à la Benjamin Button

At first, you look like a corpse
then a less dead corpse
then merely skeletal
then ninety with a little head fuzz
then eighty-ish with thinning gray strands
then a seventy-year-old man with a crew cut
then a slender, chic sixty-year-old woman
then a fine-featured lady in her fifties
then a hip forty with a dyed blond quiff
then a fit, flat-chested thirty-something
then a grad student . . .

then one day,
the first of the new semester,
a student asks what classes you're taking
without knowing you're his instructor.

This is a true story.

Blondes Have More Touching Up to Do

Having been a natural redhead all of my life,
I decide it's time for a change when my hair grows back in.

When my stylist asks what I want done
to the inch-long mousy fuzz I present him with
after having had no use of his services for over a year,
I tell him "rock star."

Thankfully, his idea of what this might look like
is exactly what I had in mind.

Otherwise I'd have had to shave it all
and start from scratch.

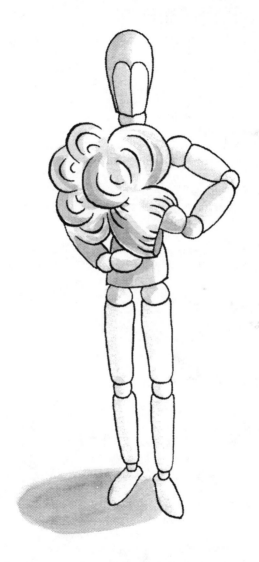

(Fill in the Blank)

Hey! You're looking great!
(for someone who has cancer)

Your hair's so long!
(compared to how long it was that year you were bald)

You've put on weight!
(that's a compliment)

How's everything?
(did the cancer go away, or what?)

The kids must be so grown-up now!
(who was going to get them if, you know . . .)

What are you up to these days?
(are you back at work?)

How's Jack?
(rumor has it he was going to leave you . . .)

Sorry I haven't been in touch—I've just been so busy.
(I avoided you like the plague)

It was so good running into you here!
   (as opposed to at your funeral)

Got to dash—say hi to Jack for me!
   (because if you two do break up, I want a shot at him)

I'll call you, we'll do lunch sometime.
   (yeah, right)

Ciao!
   (see ya, wouldn't wanna be ya)

Fill 'Er Up

Every week, my boobs get another fill up,
more saline *cc*'s to rev my chest's big engines.

The expanders have magnetic valves
which can be easily located

and stuck with a syringe the size of a turkey baster
which looks exactly as gruesome as it sounds.

You know that scene in *Pulp Fiction*
where John Travolta plunges a hypodermic

full of adrenaline into Uma Thurman's chest?
Like that. But with less bickering and sweat.

Twice.
One in each side.

I do not tire of grossing people out
by telling them this.

Pros and Cons

In the plastic surgeon's office
I hold first a saline-filled implant
and then a silicone-filled one.

Here's how to replicate the experience at home:
for the former, fill a balloon with water,
and see how it ripples and sloshes as you
palm it from hand to hand.

For the latter, reach for the nearest boob
and give it a squeeze.

(Best to ask first.)

Real Fake Boobs

For the second time in a year you wake from surgery
with your chest swathed in bandages.

This time, they've replaced the saline-filled expanders
with primo silicone implants, the Rolls-Royce of fake boobs.

The automobile reference is no accident:
you can't wait to take them for a spin.

Rack

You'd think that after getting implants,
I might refer to my chest as a "rack."

Instead, they remind me of the torture
I went through to get them.

Every week, another 50 ml stretch
expanding my vocabulary for pain.

Go Figure

When told you will lose your breasts,
one word that comes to mind is "disfigured."

But that's only if you consider your breasts
to be the principal element of your figure.

But breasts
figure

less than you think. When you get new breasts,
you become reconfigured.

Reckless

When you are dying of cancer,
putting on your seat belt
every single time
seems unnecessary.

At first, you go without it
on the ride back from
the plastic surgeon
after every saline fill-up
because it gets in the way.

You come to like hunching forward
over the wheel and discover the secret
of taking corners like a race car driver:
shifting your hips in the seat
to maintain your center of gravity.

And so what if you get pulled over?
So what if you fly through the windscreen?

For a little while you feel alive.

Once your hair has grown back
you return to old habits

and buckle up like everyone else.
You have no more excuses.

You miss that feeling
the way you miss having a nurse
whose job is to ask you how you are
at least once a week.

Eh, you say.
I'll live.

☺ ☺

The great thing about brand-new boobs
is that they're blank slates.
You can have your new nipples put
wherever you like.

The plastic surgeon sends me home
with two adhesive circles the size of areolas
with a little metal button in the center of each.

I'm to position them in the mirror.
Bang in the center?
Slightly higher?

I think about my former boobs,
sagging from years of breast-feeding,
the nipples shrugging south.

The next day, the day before surgery,
the surgeon draws around them with a black Sharpie
so she knows where to cut.

I consider turning them into smiley faces
out of sheer joy.

Dolly Parton Poem

In addition to her flaming locks of auburn hair,
ivory skin, eyes of emerald green
and voice as soft as summer rain,
Jolene probably had spectacular tits too.

But Dolly couldn't mention that.
Obviously.

Cleavage

You might be surprised to learn
that *cleavage* refers not to the breasts
but to the valley between them,

the space where they are not.
The cleavage is the cleft between two things
which cleave together and yet are cleaved apart.

A Slight Chill

As soon as the sun goes down
or the temperature dips
below sixty, it becomes clear
what else boobs are good for.

With no fat on my upper torso,
there is nothing to insulate
my chest cavity,
my heart and lungs
circulating blood

as if it's a nice rosé
being chilled for dinner.

That's Hysterical

My dodgy genes raise my chances
    of getting ovarian cancer
        slightly

Which explains why my oncologist
    keeps asking me if I'm
        getting

them removed. *It's something*
    we ought to think about, she says,
        as if I haven't.

She, of course, has, and together
    we've come to very different
        decisions.

It's best to take out the uterus too,
    just to be on the safe side,
        she says.

I wonder if I'd still be a woman
    without any of my working
        parts.

At least, if I ever got mad about it,
    no one could say I was
        hysterical.

Mixed Metaphor

Every dinnertime, you pop that little white pill
and hope it knows it's supposed to *prevent*
you getting more cancer, rather than *give* you
more cancer. Tamoxifen is, ironically,
a known carcinogen.

They discovered that the radiation
routinely prescribed to keep the cancer at bay
ends up causing heart disease down the road.

If it's not one thing, it's another.

You roll your dice and hope they come up heads.
Then you realize dice don't have heads.
They don't even have tails.
All they have is numbers, and they're just odds.
People tell you it all evens out in the end.

You hope you come up trumps.

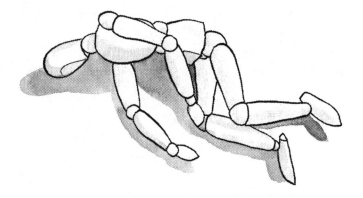

TUBE

(Totally Unnecessary Breast Exam)

There was this time I had lunch with a guy who knew I'd had cancer and had heard that I'd gotten implants, and he didn't stop staring at them the entire time. When he was saying goodbye, he suddenly reached out with both hands and squeezed them. It was like a cartoon. He took his time about it. I suddenly understood that the entire lunch was, for him, in aid of this very moment. *Thanks*, he said, when he was done. He seemed satisfied with his exploration. I don't think I said anything at all.

Estrogen Elegy

At first, all you can think about
is the one big loss,
the thing they will cut off
and pick apart
and throw away
that you will not be buried with—

but it turns out
that loss doesn't just apply
to things that can be removed
with a scalpel.
Cancer is a cascade
of unfolding losses
that only begins with the blade.

The things you will miss the most
cannot be held in the palm of your hand.
How much does your estrogen weigh?
How much your desire?

O Tamoxifen, little white pill
half as big as the tumor they found
that I swallow daily like a prayer,
does what you might give me
equal what you take away?

Stuck Like Glue

I hate it when people say
"We survivors have to stick together!"

Why?
Because we're so good at falling apart?

Or is there some awful side effect
I haven't encountered yet?

Chica Chica Boom Chic

In my quest never to become complacent
about learning new things,
or thinking that I'm too old to do so,
I take up guitar.

By "take up," I mean I pick one up
and try to get my fingers into the right shapes
to make chords.

But there's an obstacle
I hadn't counted on: my right boob.

There it sits, between me and the guitar
like a grapefruit strapped to my chest.
I can't hoist it up and it won't squash flat.

No wonder Carmen Miranda wore them on her head.

Victoria's Secret

I never liked wearing a bra
when I had to. First, it was to hide
any evidence of nipple under a T-shirt.
Then, for support.

Now, I have discovered what
Victoria's *real* secret is:
the only thing a bra is for is packaging.

That's why they have bows.

Pull Yourself Up by Your Brastraps

Cancer survivors are insufferable.

They're always telling people how awful
it was, relishing the chance to share
a battle story meant to scare the bejesus
out of you, without thinking that
you might, at this very minute,
have cancer too and not even know it.

See what I mean?

Punctuation

The chemo dashes you right into menopause

without so much as a comma.
Everything that grows from a follicle dies,
and that includes the tiny eggs from ovaries,
petering out like so many ellipses . . .

. . . taking with them the monthly ebb and flow of
the sentence that is your life and replacing it
with chaos, hot flashes and night sweats,
as if the chemo itself wasn't bad enough.

A year goes by without so much as a period,
which if truth be told, you miss.
Then one day it returns and just like that
you make sense again, you flow.

The oncologist is shocked—she never sees this.
I'm only forty-one. Still, you know what they say:
no surprise for the writer, no surprise for the reader.
My future is no longer a question.

I have become an exclamation mark.

Beating Around the Bush

I always expected the "change of life"
to happen when everything else changed
—when gray hairs and wrinkles appeared—
which is to say, much later on.

But chemo throws you into menopause
immediately, so that in addition to the many
physical degradations you have to get used to,
you have hot flashes and night sweats too.

It's not until you lose "vaginal elasticity"
that you realize you even had it to begin with.
The only remedies are hormonal treatments
(not an option) and regular sex
(good luck with that).

That leaves the next best thing:
what used to be called "marital aids,"
but which nowadays are given actual names,
possibly in homage to the well,
and extremely well-endowed fellows
they are modeled after.

Such things can be prescribed by a doctor
and purchased from your local pharmacist

if the thought of buying one anonymously
on the internet is too daunting a prospect.

If I tell you I have a hot date with "Carlos,"
believe me when I say I'm just doing it for my health.

Killing Time

When people say
"I can't wait for this day to be over"
I cringe.

You Lose Some, You Win Some

Unlike some chick in a romance novel,
I never could come from nipple stimulation.
Or come much, at all.
Now, I'll never get the chance.

That's OK; all those lost nerves relocated,
like snowbirds, south.
They sing and sing and sing
the sweetest song.

The C-Word

We stumble and trip over the words,
not knowing whether I *have* cancer
or *had* cancer

and is it *the* cancer
or *my* cancer
or *a* cancer

or just IT?

And is IT in remission
or gone or still somewhere
ready to light up an MRI
like a city at night
when seen from a plane?

Cured begins with a *C* too.
I decide I'll just go ahead and call myself that.

Dream Lover

for Matthew

When I'm with him,
I forget about the scars.
He says *I'm holding your breasts*,
even though I can't tell he's doing so.

He calls them *breasts*.
That's all they are.

I'm hungry once again.

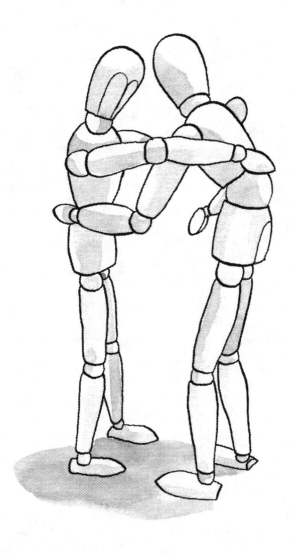

Coda

Last night I dreamed I was breast-feeding a baby—one of mine, though which I can't say, as they are all grown now—the way one does several months into the process. That is to say, lying down. I leaned over, and guided my nipple, swollen and engorged, into the waiting baby's eager mouth, and it clamped on and sucked. Any mother who has nursed will be familiar with the sweet relief this brings to the rock-hard breast as it releases its milk. The trouble is I no longer have any breasts, having lost them to cancer years ago. But I woke up with a smile, happy to have been, for that short sublunary time, whole again.

Those who have never lost a limb cannot know, except as a stretch of the imagination, what it is like to experience the disarming sensation of having a phantom one. It's not just something that affects those recently afflicted, either; it can creep up many years afterwards, in a dream, say, when the brain draws from a deep well of sense memory that predates the loss. Just like the surprising appearance of those people one has not seen or even thought about in years—as real as can be in your dream—you can appear as your former self, using that lost limb.

When we talk about amputation, we usually think first of those wounded in military action, or perhaps car accidents, who have suffered the loss of a leg or an arm. We imagine how it must be to use a prosthetic or a wheelchair, and marvel at those who have mastered mechanical substitutes to pursue their physical activities, such as runners on springy feet. We wonder how someone with a mechanical arm can scratch themselves, and what on earth those who've lost both arms do to—well, masturbate.

The intimate questions get lost in the shuffle. After all, it's more important to be able to get from A to B or to make yourself a cup of coffee or to type on a computer or brush your hair. Going to the toilet, bathing, sex—it doesn't bear thinking about. But these are ambulatory concerns. What about those whose amputation has been of something unseen and therefore flies under the radar? Millions of women have had their breasts amputated due to cancer, but even if they have been replaced with implants, the tissue is still missing, the silicone mounds still utterly numb.

I might look "normal," but my sensation ends where my ribs do, flat as a boy's. The implants have no feeling, no response to cold, cannot tell me if they are being touched by a curious passerby. I am glad to have them, even if they look like two halves of a grapefruit, a little (OK, a lot) too perky for a woman my age. After breast-feeding two babies, my own breasts were beginning to look somewhat older than the rest of me when they got the chop.

In fact, I was still feeding my son, who was as slow to wean as I was reluctant to give up that particular intimacy of motherhood. The last thing I did, prepped in my surgical cap and gown, was stand over the sink in the OR bathroom and express the last of my milk with my fingers, squeezing out what seemed, at the time, all that remained of my womanhood. The thin sharp jets hit the stainless steel with a hiss. I looked once in the mirror, willing my mind to be blank, to begin the process of disassociation with a part of me that would soon be gone. I said goodbye to them, and thanks, and climbed on the gurney.

When you are diagnosed with breast cancer, you enter an abrupt flurry of activity and emotion, which culminates a short time later in something being cut off or out, and usually, many months of toxic treatment in the form of chemotherapy and radiation. Your life as you knew it simply stops. Nothing can prepare you for the mental challenge of a voluntary amputation. It's not like having an accident and the next thing you know, you're waking up in recovery with bandages, someone having to tell you what you no longer have. One is not any less horrifying than the other. With breast cancer—as with any planned surgery— you have time to think about it beforehand. You have to walk into that room.

But among all the mountains of information you wade through prior to surgery, there is nothing that really tells you how to prepare for not having breasts. While puberty gives you time to adjust to a new center of gravity and shape, surgery returns you to a boyish figure all of a sudden, and takes with it the sexuality of the top half of your body. It becomes necessary to learn how to compensate for this—and you can, and do. One of the biggest motivators in my decision to get a reconstruction wasn't to bring the sexy back, however—it was to give my young children something familiar to cuddle up to. Having become used to their using my chest for comfort, I couldn't imagine my children not needing to use me that way.

This book is a reflection of the attitude I brought to the healing process, and which I believe helped me make the transition from one kind of body—and one kind of worldview—to another, of the kind that surviving cancer makes a necessity. I decided early on to see the humor in my situation, to laugh in the face of fear. My chemo nurse once confided in me, as I reached the end of my punishing regime of treatment, that she could tell who was going to be OK by how capable they were of laughing, especially at themselves. To find joy in life when life seems so precarious a proposition is to win, no matter what. I don't think having cancer is funny. But I do find the absurdities it throws your way something to smile at. The smile says "I've been there, get that."

Any day now, my children will decide they no longer want to climb into my bed in their pj's and cuddle at dawn. They can only just remember that time Mummy had no hair and was so sick. Forgetting is a blessing. I draw them close and remember everything *else*.

Acknowledgments

I would like to thank the following people, whose care, friendship, love, and support was, and continues to be, invaluable:

Barbara Burridge, Mike Myers, Toni Myers, Roger Burridge, Patricia Burridge, Jay Burridge, Cody Burridge, Jackson Myers, Paul Myers, Rick Myers, Lucia Judy, Javier Judy, Matthew Schmidt, Tim Pryse-Hawkins, Stephen Curtis, Bernard Gibbes, Bill Kirchner, Chuck Kinder, Mark Weber, Gerry Locklin, Barbara Kauffman, Aimee Beal, Elaine Leggett, Jonna Hall, Nurse Carol, and doctors Michael Finikiotis, Donald Keenan, Carolyn De La Cruz, and Pryia Rastogi.

And to these lovely people without whose professional guidance and assistance this book would not have been:

Sarah Funke Butler (for finding and believing in me), Sarah Knight (for being a brilliantly perceptive editor), and Les Kay (for supplying a kick-ass subtitle).

The following poems have appeared in these wonderful places, sometimes in a different form:

"Hospital-Grade Benadryl," *New Plains Review*
"Telling It Like It Is," *Nerve Cowboy*
"You Can Never Be Too Rich or Too Thin?" *Nerve Cowboy*
"No Such Thing as a Free Lunch," *Pittsburgh Post-Gazette*

A shorter version of this book was a finalist in the *Nerve Cowboy* Chapbook Contest. Thank you to the editors for championing my work.

About the Author

MICKI MYERS is an award-winning artist and writer originally from England. For the last twenty-five years she has lived in Pittsburgh, where she teaches English and raises her children. She maintains a number of blogs and is a regular contributor of book reviews and commentary in print. Her first book, *Trigger Finger*, won the Pearl Poetry Prize. Learn more on her website www.mickimyers.com or follow her on Twitter @mickimyers.

Printed in the United States
By Bookmasters